Parent-Practitioner Partnership

By D. M. Devine

Table of Contents

Wherever the practice of medicine is loved

So is the art of Humanity.

~Hippocarities

This book is dedicated to my husband for sharing in this journey of parenthood with me and to each of my 3 children who have taught me a great deal about life, love and about myself. Our first son taught us lessons in faith, our daughter taught us lessons in joy and our youngest son taught us the lessons in hope.

Every day you each show me what it is to be a hero.

I would also like to recognize the wonderful practitioners who we have formed lasting partnerships with. These are the people who exemplify these practices for me and excel in the practice of medicine simply by being who they are and sharing themselves and their gifts with us. They are family friends, incredible people and are each partially responsible for the fact that we are alive and healthy today.

Gerard Vockley, MD

Stephen Kurachek, MD

David Schmeling, MD

Cheryl Hanson, MD

Beth Gillis, MD

Barry Barudin, MD

Introduction

This is not an introduction to the concepts of the book but rather a brief introduction and background on me, the writer. I have been an educator for well over a decade now and feel strongly that it is important to know a little about the teacher and where the information is coming from before absorbing the knowledge into your beliefs.

My husband and I have a great deal of experience with health care providers in our time as parents. We had our 3 children in 3 years, not a practice I would recommend, although it is far more stress for the parents than for the kids.

For our first son we learned the devastating lesson on how to make end of life decisions, when he was born without kidneys and died as an infant. His life was a brief gift of love that we still cherish to this day. Our 17-year-old daughter's birth was literally a 'walk into paradise' and continues to be that through the years of watching her grow, find her passions and achieve amazing things. She had some trouble briefly as an infant but is now 'the picture of health', "knock on wood" or whatever it is one does to ensure this continues. Our 16-year-old son has multiple complicated health issues. He was born blind and mute, and with very delayed myelination across his entire brain surface. We were told that he: would never see, speak, know us, sit, crawl or stand. To date he: sees, speaks, reads, drives a go-cart, plays baseball, love music and has an opinion on everything! He has taught us more in his 15 years than I ever imagined I would come to learn in a lifetime. He still teaches us the meaning of hope, love and patience every day.

Our journey into the wild wonderful world of parenthood was not easy for us in other ways. I had complicated pregnancies, lost an organ for each of the first 2 and had a stroke in the sixth month of my last pregnancy. When I was 6 months pregnant with our youngest I learned that I had a rare (less than 2 dozen people in the world) genetic disorder that is untreatable and terminal. By the time our youngest child was 4 years old I was given 3 months left to live. However, that was almost 12 years ago now and I am still going strong.

Each of our children have been a wonderful blessing and a great teacher for us. We have learned a lot and loved a lot and intend to continue on this same path for many years to come.

So, as parents, we have learned about making end-of-life decisions and lifesaving decisions. Both can be equally difficult and equally stressful. Seldom are decisions ever straightforward or simple. This is the main thrust behind the importance of discovering a healthcare provider that you can build a strong working relationship with, based upon mutual respect and shared goals.

Our family has seen over 127 doctors in the first 7 years after of our parenting, from Residents to Attendings, Surgeons to Specialists. We have worked with county facilities, small partnerships and some of our nation's largest healthcare venues. The ideas in this book apply to any type of healthcare practitioner at any type of facility. The concepts are really designed to guide you through the process of using your own instincts and preferences.

Professionally I have worked in various aspects of medicine all of my adult life. I have a Master's Degree in Adult Education specializing in Medical Education. I am also a licensed Parent Educator. I have written medical curriculum, assisted in the orientation process of residents and medical student at a major metropolitan hospital and sat on a committee to design a pediatric patient-centered care unit. I have also sat on a parent advisory committee at one of the country's largest medical centers for several years hoping to be instrumental in upgrading their policies in Family Centered Care.

If you feel lost already by some of the terminology that I am using, assure yourself that basically my professional goals is to make sure the healthcare team is up to the challenge of Family Centered Care so when you are out 'shopping' for your healthcare provider there will be people out there ready, willing, and able to work with you as a team and sincerely value your input and expertise as a parent.

We are facing a time of great fluctuation and enormous challenges in healthcare delivery. The country is experiencing growing pains within the medical world and many of the responsibilities that were once shouldered by the practitioner are now placed squarely in the lap of the patient. If you hear people refer to patients as consumers, this is a valid form of reference. No longer are we matched with a lifelong practitioner, we are now required to shop, investigate, interview and select our healthcare team. Take this responsibility seriously, especially in this role for your child's welfare. Although you may now have a healthy child and you may rarely see a practitioner your circumstances may change in an instant and you will be thankful that you did your

research and referrals now rather than in the face of

a medical emergency. Decisions are better made

with a cool head, time and investigation. Use this

book as a tool to educate, advice and empower you

to jump head first into this challenging, yet rewarding

responsibility.

Welcome to the Wonderful World of Medicine

There are two things that are vital to understand when beginning your journey into the medical world as a parent. First it is important that you know the role a practitioner should provide in the healthcare team. It is my firm belief that a practitioner should use their vast knowledge of medicine to listen, educate, and then empower families to make an informed decision about their child's; care, treatment, diagnosis, on-going plan, care delivery team, and families level of involvement. It is important to understand my assumption of the practitioner's role throughout this book and throughout my life in medicine. I consider our physicians to be valuable members of our health care team when they are knowledgeable of their craft but respectful of our different levels of involvement. Never forget that like the old adage about a ham and egg breakfast: The pig and the chicken had different levels of involvement. The chicken was 'involved' but the pig was committed! This is true for the different degrees of involvement between a health practitioner and a parent. The practitioner is involved but the parent is committed. A parent takes the child home, lives with and loves them 24 hours a day 7 days a week. A parent's life is entirely wrapped up in the investment they hold in their child's health and happiness.

The second role to be defined and understood is the role of the parent in the health care delivery team. Talk with your parents, grandparents and elderly relatives about their relationship with their child's physician, or better yet, just sit back and listen. The first role in parenting, as most of you already know is, "advice getter." No matter what your child's age is and no matter if you have a PhD. in childrearing you still get the gift of endless advice, stories, adages and tall tales. After you listen to your loved ones' advice explaining how they believe you should secure a good physician and then just sit back to let them do their work. For most grandparents, this was the reality of a parent physician relationship when their children were growing up. Statements like: 'Trust them to make all the best decisions.' were common and heart felt. Then before you leap ahead, remember the only catch here is that healthcare is entirely different now then it was even 20 years ago. These variations are as vast as how and where hospitals are located; to who reimburses for what care. There are stacks and stacks of political rationale as to the form and function for each of these practices but in the end one of the greatest things that affects lay-people on a daily basis is the demand that doctors are now under to see more, do more, know more and do it all in 10 minutes, while seeing 40 patients in a single day. These massive requirements transfer the role for the parent from receiver to active participant. Parents are now students looking to gain knowledge, champions for their child's desires, and advocates hoping to improve their child's daily health. So when a relative asks why you are asking questions of a health care provider, feel confident in your role as medical advocate, this is now a job qualification for any newly applying parent.

#1. Medicine is NOT an exact Science
It is an Art form

"Each person is a variation
Whose difference is so profound
that no scientist could
study or memorize them all."

This is important for people to understand so that

they are aware that there are choices, no longer

single answers. Historically, medicine was more of a

single choice option. You were diagnosed with an

illness and then prescribed a medication to treat that

illness. However, medicine in the 21st century offers

many treatment options, multiple timeframes and

various mindsets. This allows you the wonderful gift

of options. If medicine was simply studying the

problem and then matching it with its proven

treatment there would be no mystery; nor any

miracles either. There are currently thousands of categorized medical diagnoses yet only a handful; actually have a **single** proven treatment option. For all the other disorders, pains, diagnoses and disabilities there are options for exploration.

Remember that like all other forms of art, there are as many different ways to express an emotion, as there are people out there. So your goal is to find the artist, (or health care practitioner), as the case may be, that matches your level of emotional expression.

An easier way to think of this is: consider that there are doctors who simply like to make decisions; if you are one of those parents who does not want to make a choice or be involved in the decision making aspects of your child's care this would be a good partner for you. If you are overwhelmed by the complexities of the decision's you are facing and are looking to have the puzzles solved by someone else; seek out these types of physicians or healthcare practices. These specific practices are defined as being: physician-lead institutions. Ironically these types of institutions are going away fairly quickly, because more and more patients and their families, no longer want to turn over the decisions to their practitioners. Plus as there continues to be a greater diversity of care options many families are interested in exploring the choices.

So if you are a patient or family member that is interested in partnering with a care provider who sees their role as a member of a larger healthcare delivery team. A practitioner who is interested in diagnosing and then defining the treatment options along with the risks and benefits of each. If you are looking to be a valued member of your child's health care delivery team you may wish to seek out a practitioner interested in partnering with you. These practitioners will help to grow and develop the team of providers that will give work together to meet your treatment goals. For instance, Physical Therapists, Occupational Therapists, Alternative Medicine Providers, Social Workers, teachers, nutritionists and holistic providers are now understood to be valuable members of the care delivery team. The few Physician-driven institutions still practice in the old style of placing the doctor on a pedestal instead on as an equal member of the team. I am sure after reading this description you can discern why physician-lead institutions are fading fast, and why the patient's that have the strongest draw this this style of medicine come from the elderly community. Since many patients from those eras are still most comfortable in physician lead way of practicing medicine.

For all other patients who are looking to explore their various treatment options with guidance you need to find a practitioner who can provide direction and advice while still respecting your final decision. It is vitally important for you to find the practitioner who fits your values and interests. There are practitioners who are very homeopathic in their choices of treatment, if you are a parent who believes in this form of medicine find a similar practitioner. Many parents would prefer nutritional options, herbal supplements or alternative health elections to be explored before utilizing more invasive treatment options.

There are practitioners who wish to educate you about your options and then allow you to make the final decision. If you wish to be an important part of your child's healthcare team; seek out these physicians.

The differences don't even need to be this extreme. You may be more aggressive or less. You may believe strongly in pharmaceutical intervention or you may be a person who refuses to take medicine when you have a headache. You may opt to cut something out if it gives you problems where others may be slow to choose surgical intervention.

This is a time, like many others in your future as a parent; that you must listen to your instincts, ask many questions and then go the way of your heart and mind. These two things are usually your very best leaders. Spend time up front meeting with and interviewing a variety of care providers so that you have a strong partner and advocate along your child's health journey.

Practitioners who succeed in this new medical world of partnering are those who listen to, watch, trust, and respect their patients. Each person is a variation whose difference is so profound that no scientist could study or memorize them all. This is why doctors should look to you for the answers to their questions about individual variations, wants, lifestyle preferences and not the other way around. You also hold the answers to the questions of your child and the path he/she will take. We have had a few wonderful examples of this in our own lives. Our youngest son was born with a very rare genetic disorder that caused him to be blind. Of course everyone assumed that he would never see. Yet by his 3rd birthday they up-graded him to cortically blind, which simply means that the structures of your eyes seem to be intact and working but your brain cannot seem to process the information which still leaves you unable to see. By the time he was 4 years old he had totally graduated out of the blindness program at school, a feat that had never happened before. So imagine when we see a new practitioner and casually mention that our son was blind but he can see fine now. It takes a strong practitioner to be mindful of all the things they learned in medical school and still believe in the amazing power of the human spirit to overcome incredible odds. We find some practitioners who can stretch in their thinking and some who choose not to look beyond what a textbook claims to be impossible. We have learned early on that we need to find practitioners who can set aside their textbook learning and embrace a larger reality. This is where the art of healing takes over when the science is learning new concepts.

The best time to begin looking for a primary care provider is during your pregnancy or if you move communities. Oftentimes clinics will set up appointments for expectant parents to come and meet a provider.

Another way to begin your exploration to find a physician partner is to ask friends, co-workers and other doctors for referrals before proceeding with an initial interview. But don't simply inquire about which practitioner they use. Instead make sure to ask them why they liked him/her, what types of problems did they turn to them for diagnosis and how was that handled? Investigate as to how the diagnosis was achieved. Were they as parents asked to be intimately involved in the care-delivery team? Ask about how often drugs where given for treatment and in what framework were they turned to. How was communication handled within that clinic setting? How long do you typically wait for an appointment and then how long do you wait when you arrive at the clinic? You need to explore an extensive background of experiences before you can opt to pursue this referral. Oftentimes one person will really connect with a practitioner and then another will find them to be too domineering or too passive, so it is not enough to simply seek a referral. Make sure to practice this when looking for a specialist as well, it is often more important to have a working partnership with a surgeon or specialist because they will need to guide you in some difficult decisions.

Within the framework of this newly formed partnership there must be mutual respect and a great deal of trust. For these concepts to develop it works best over a period of time for maturation of the relationship. One key way for this to happen is to make a specific point to pick a practitioner and then stick with them. I know that this concept is easy to write but very difficult to achieve. Many times you call in when your child is sick and your practitioner is booked out for several weeks. It is important to put your child's health first in this instance and see whoever is available, but you can also mention that you would like to be called if your practitioner has a cancellation. You can also schedule a routine follow-up with your primary care physician at a later date to discuss the outcome of the decisions made and ask specific questions. All of this seems to be taxing and wasted time, but a single strep throat may become a repeated problem and physicians can deal with patients much better if they have a running history of the difficulty and if they also feel knowledgeable about the child's auxiliary health. You are building a daily relationship by sharing your families' functioning both in times of crisis and in times of calm. Most physicians will tell you that they have a much easier time treating and following established patients for the simple reason that they feel confident in their relationship with the patient's caregivers' abilities and have a knowledge base of their requirements and desires.

#2. You Know Your Child Like No One Else

"...We are in a 50/50 partnership.
You hold 50% of the knowledge by understanding diseases
processes, diagnosis and treatment options. I hold 50% of the
knowledge because I am the expert on my child's needs."

This makes you an intrical partner in any healthcare team that makes treatment choices for your child. You hold the answers to the mystery of your child's individual abilities, idiosyncrasies and emotional capabilities. One of my best examples for this one is our son's NEED to be with us as soon as he comes out of anesthesia. Our first visit to a distant hospital for one of his surgeries turned into an interesting, and now in retrospect funny illustrations of this. We told the surgeons that we would probably need to be brought back as quick as they could after the procedure or our little guy had ways of getting us back there when he needed us. Of course they smiled, shook their heads and explained that they would come for us as soon as he was actually waking up. We were sitting in the waiting area and had just gotten the update by phone that the surgery was wrapping up when we saw a person in full surgical scrubs running down the hall while we heard the overhead page for a pediatric code. We didn't hesitate. We knew they were coming for us. Our inventive little man screamed so hard the minute he had the tube out of his throat that he held his breath and coded. In the end the surgeons apologized and realized that when we said NEEDED US we weren't kidding.

It doesn't take long for a parent to learn the subtle and not-so-subtle clues that your child gives off to let you know how they are feeling. You know if she/he is acting different from their norm or if they are having a slightly odd reaction to a drug. You know if they are sleeping more than what is typical for them. Be confident in your knowledge when you face a doctor who is telling you what is going to happen to your child. No one should ever TELL YOU what treatment is planned for your child. Even if that treatment is as simple as whether or not to give antibiotics when the physician finds a pink eardrum. You need to be confident in your role as decision maker for your child. This does not mean that you should override the physician's knowledge of medical treatment, it simply means that you must follow your instincts about your child's welfare and encourages your physician to offer all the options.

Each treatment option should be thoroughly explained to you, pros & cons, side effects, what happens if you opt for no treatment and any long-term concerns? In the case of the pink eardrum your questions may include; what are the benefits/harms of antibiotics? Should we wait a couple of days and see if it is a virus that will run its course without drug intervention? Are there any other signs I should be watching for? Once you have the answers to your concerns and the doctor has explained your options, it is at this point that your medical staff should step back and give you the time and power to make appropriate decisions as a family. Now I know that many of you are laughing at me and thinking "In a perfect world", but it really should be like this and if you do not feel that you are getting that option at your present clinic speak up, ask more questions, clearly state your willingness to learn and when all else fails: never hesitate to seek practitioners elsewhere. You are the consumer of your care. Look for it, review it, educate yourself, and then decide.

Make sure to utilize all of the staff at your healthcare facility. Although doctors, nurses and medical staff have great requirements for their time; most went in to medicine for the sole purpose to help people. If your practitioner is unable to spend enough time with you for your comfort level, ask if there is an education department or if it is possible to receive additional information in the form of pamphlets, videos, or reference material that you could review on your own time before contacting the practitioner to decide upon treatment options. Utilize public libraries and reference materials to educate yourself about the disorder/disease and to help formulate questions to pose at your next visit. Don't be afraid to ask the nurse who rooms you if there are others resources out there for information. Utilize your pharmacist for information about drug treatments. Ask other parents about their experiences with this diagnosis. Many times your best resource is simply talking to your friends; you may find someone who knows someone who was in a similar situation. A wonderful example of this came when our son had a G-tube placed in his stomach for feeding needs. We talked with the nurse, the surgeon, the surgical resident, and friends but it wasn't until I spoke with our friend who works in special education that I got valuable insight. She offered me a parent to contact who had been in a similar situation. There was no amount of structured medical training that could replace the insight and hands-on knowledge that parenting a child with a G-tube offered. She was able to share with us the daily struggles faced with a G-tube. She opened my eyes to the concerns never mentioned by the medical staff but also helped us to see hope and adaptations that would improve my child's overall life quality. One simple one I remember was: when a G-tube is inserted your child will have a difficult time wearing clothes with a waistband. This was a basic bit of information that helped us take an active role in helping our child by having enough forethought to have purchased a wardrobe of one-piece outfits.

There are many resources out there for you if you expend the time and energy to investigate. The unfortunate thing is that when you are facing many of these issues you are too overwhelmed by daily cares to have any 'extra' time. Often the time best spent is time on the internet searching for resources based on a disease, diagnosis or treatment. I have found great success searching for an area Children's hospital and then looking at their resource center or many have a listing of helpful 'approved' websites where you can feel confident of the information you will be receiving. Some diagnoses are large enough that you can find an association affiliated with it (i.e. diabetes, asthma, cystic fibrosis, epilepsy etc.) You can do a simple search for the disease name and then more specific searches once you find the site. These sites are often great resources for the newest treatments options, facilities that specialize in them etc. If you do not have access to the internet at home many public library systems have computers available to the public for free use. I also found that both pediatric hospitals that we use have computers available for family use and they each have huge Parent

Resource centers and are more than happy to assist you in your search of information.

There may be other times when you are confident in your practitioner's ability to decide on procedures and treatments. But no matter how the decision is reached you should always feel confident in the fact that if you would ever choose to disagree or ask for more information your practitioner would respect your need for a greater understanding and encourage you to seek a second opinion.

At any time in your relationship with your child's physician you should feel confident that you could say; "We are in a 50/50 partnership. You hold 50% of the knowledge by understanding diseases processes, diagnosis and treatment options. I hold 50% of the knowledge because I am the expert on my child's needs. We each need the other's input in order to make the right decision for my child." If you smirk when you read that and do not feel that it describes your current parent-physician partnership you should discuss this with your practitioner.

So if you can accept these statements about your healthcare relationship as fact before even approaching the healthcare setting. The next step is to review the 4 vital concepts for making your relationship successful and hopefully helping to ensure proper care of your child. Try to always keep one goal in mind: Optimal care for your child.

The concepts that I feel are most valuable when working within a health care team I have divided up into 4 categories: Be Accurate, Be Honest, Ask Questions and Leave with an Agreed upon Plan. Each of these concepts has important subsets where you will see the overall value of the concept. If you equip yourself with confidence in your mission and know that you are following a set path it will help to alleviate the stress that is usually wrapped up in seeking care.

Concept #1
Be Accurate

Knowledge is Power!

It is very important that you have an accurate and up-to-date report on your child's health status any time that you seek medical advice. There are many reasons for this but one of the most important is that knowledge is power. Often times you are afraid to speak up because you aren't really sure if that was the medicine that caused such bad diaper rash or how many ear infections has your child really had in the last 6 months. You simply know that it was disturbing enough to concern you. Yet when the practitioner starts asking you specific questions you are not certain enough to be confident. Carrying your child's medical information with you will give you that confidence.

I'm not talking about making a copy of their chart, although be aware that you do own the information in your child's health records, so if at any time you do wish to have a copy of your child's chart do not be shy about asking for it. They do have the right to charge copying fees but they DO NOT have the right to deny you a copy. You can even get original films and scans if you are moving or transferring facilities or would simply like having your own copy to bring along for second opinions or to show other specialists. A more inexpensive way to do this is to have the new facility generate a request for release of information. This way you usually by-pass all of the copying fees which can be rather spendy if your child has a large chart or you are getting copies of multiple scans. If you have the facility get the old records you just call the main clinic/hospital number, (usually medical records is the area that generates the request) but if you tell the main desk that you have charts or films from different facilities and would like them to be available for your physician to consult when you have your appointment they will then send you a consent form and then they will process the request for you.

It is helpful for your new physician or specialist but it is also beneficial for your child as well, because having the films, results and past studies available may save your child from repetitive testing that can be painful and costly. This is just one more reason to keep good records so that you know what tests your child has already had, when and where so you are able to collect all necessary information to assist your subsequent practitioners in making the best well-informed decisions they can.

Tips on keeping accessible & accurate medical data for each of your children.

- Start by purchasing a small spiral notebook, one that fits into your purse or back pocket. I have one for each child and have found it to be a lifesaver on more than one occasion. I have even gone so far as to use masking tape to make tabs on the side.

- It takes a little while to compile the information but once you have it in one spot it is very easy to use for reference. The notebook will become invaluable.

- I use the following headings, leaving several pages between each new heading.

- Vital Statistics
  - Child's personal info
    - Child's full name

- Child's home address and phone number
- Child's social security number
- Name of parents and/or guardians
- Parent's addresses (work and home) and phone numbers
- Child's birth date and birth place
- Emergency Numbers and contact information
  - **Allergies**

1. **Include medication allergies**
   - **If your child is allergic to one type of medication be sure to call a pharmacy and ask if there are other medications that your child should not have or other concerns related to this allergy**

2. **Make sure to include any food/pet allergies**

3. **Also Include any allergies or reactions to specific substances like Latex, bee stings and how these concerns are addressed in the event of exposure**

- Clinic Information (leave several extra pages in case you move you can use a new page to update this information. But do not discard old clinic information; I simply fold down that page in the notebook. You will always need to know all of the places your child has doctored in case there are complications down the road.)

  1. Clinic name
  2. Child's chart number
  3. Phone number and address
  4. Practitioner's full name
  5. Hospital of preference or for insurance coverage (if you have one)

- Insurance Information (leave several pages in case there are changes in your insurance information and remember to always save the outdated information as well)

  1. Child's insurance information
  2. Include the address of the company and 800

     number
  3. Make sure to list group number and policy number
  4. Policy holder information
- Birth Information
  1. Birth weight
  2. Birth length
  3. Head circumference
  4. Type of delivery (Cesarean, vaginal)
  5. Place of delivery (Home, hospital etc.)

6.   Apgar scores (if you have them, there should be 2: one a minute after delivery and one five minutes after delivery)

7.   Complications during pregnancy or delivery

• Growth (this will become invaluable if you notice a trend in your child's growth pattern that is concerning. Keep in mind that growth charts are simply a comparison of your child's growth to that of the "average" child of this age and should not be alarming if your child is in a very low or high percentile unless there are other reasons for concern.)

1.   Several pages to note ongoing growth (write these

down each time you go to a doctor's visit)

2.   It is nice to include the child's percentile

3.   Weight & date

4.   Height & date

5.   Head circumference & date

6.   Chest circumference & date

- Vital Characteristics

    1.   Identifying birth marks

    2.   Hair color (make sure to note major changes as

          time goes by)

    3.   Eye color (note changes after child has hit their first birthday)

    4.   Any variations in their physical appearance.

    5.   Birth marks or identifying scars

- Dental records

    1.   When baby teeth appeared (I often just draw an open mouth and draw in the teeth as they come)

2. Then I mark when they were lost

3. And finally when adult teeth replaced them.

4. Any dental hardware currently in place

- Vaccination record

    1. Make sure to include that date each vaccination was given,

    2. Where it was given

    3. The form it was given in (i.e. Shot, liquid etc.)

    4. If the child had any problems or reactions to the vaccine

- Practitioners/Specialists

    1. Practitioner's name

    2. Clinic Address

    3. Phone number

    4. Type of medicine they specialize in

- Lists of Tests and Procedures that your child has had

1.   Name of Procedure

2.   Date and Place where it was done

3.   It is also nice to include a small description of the

        procedure and how your child responded to it

- Surgeries

1.   Name of the procedure (go on-line to look for correct spelling or look at the consent form)

2.   Hospitals where they had it

3.   Address & general phone number

4.   All the doctors who participated in their care (It helps a great deal to get the name of the anesthesiologist who performed the surgery in case you need or want to return to them for reference or to use them for additional surgeries)

5.   Dates of surgery and length of admission

6.   Any problems or complications.

- Family history. Things that are good to include in this section is whether or not you have a family history of: (for each item make sure to include the name of the person who suffers from it and how they are related to the child. I.e. maternal grandmother, Lisa Smith) It is important for you to note this information yourself. Once you have children of your own you shouldn't rely on asking your parents "What disease did Uncle Bob have, I never can remember?" This becomes timely and cumbersome if there is an emergency situation and you need to contact relatives to find out if there is a prominent bleeding disorder in your family's immediate history. It is also nice to have them written down as you usually need this information in high stress situations which is often when the name is most likely to slip your mind.

1.   High Blood Pressure

2.   High Cholesterol

3.   Diabetes

4.   Heart problems

5.   Early blindness

6.   Early death

7.   Mental retardation/Neurological

disorders

8.   Arthritis

9.   Bleeding Disorders

10.   Problems with Anesthesia

11.   Genetic Malformations

12.   Other

- Medications that your child has taken and any

problems that

he/she has had with them. (Leave blank

pages here as well because they may

develop problems as they age.)

- I leave many pages at the back

where you write down questions.

You may choose to use these question pages to jot down things that are not significant enough to call doctor immediately, but something you may wish to inquire about at your next visit. For my son, who has multiple specialists, I write each specialty on the top of a page and as things come up specific to that doctor I jot it down. Then when I get to the office I am equipped with what I need to ask instead of sitting there thinking; 'I know I wanted to ask you something...' Typically right when I get home is when I remember, and then I have the task of trying to get back in touch with them.

The next important part of keeping good records is writing down when medications were given. When your child gets sick and you begin to give medications for fever or other symptoms make sure to have a sheet of paper taped to the refrigerator or bathroom mirror where you note the time, date and medication you gave. This serves many important functions. The most important is when you get up in the middle of the night with a child you seldom have a strong recollection of the time, thus it is exceedingly easy to administer medications too closely spaced together which can be life threatening. The other reason for these notations is if you later realize that the problem is escalating and you decide to take the child to the emergency room, you will need to know the exact time and types of medications that you have given in the last 24 hours. An easy way to do this is to take a piece of construction paper and make a blank chart listing the medications that you frequently administer. Then laminate the piece of paper and attach it to the back of the medicine cabinet door with a string holding a crayon. The reason for this set-up is that the crayon will wipe right off the laminated paper and it will be a set method of notation so that all of the caregivers will easily remember to utilize this method whenever sicknesses are encountered.

Example:

Insulin	Date & time given	Allergy Meds	Date & Time give

My favourite way to keep track of when you give medications, especially for medications which are given infrequently and only for illness or pain; Like Tylenol, Motrin, Cough Syrup etc. You probably don't have a laminated sheet on the refrig when your child turns up with a fever at 2 a.m. and if you are like me;

enjoy getting as much sleep as possible, you won't

be printing off a sheet to make notes on at 2 a.m.

Here is a creative answer to all of your problems in 3

easy steps:

WHEN MEDICATIONS ARE GIVEN

Always keep medications in the same bathroom so that you have a universal spot where everyone has to come to in order to get the medications. This solves many problems like: mom waking up at 1 a.m. going to the upstairs bathroom giving a dose of acetaminophen then falling asleep. Baby wakes again at 2 a.m. Mom is so tired she doesn't even wake up so dad wakes up feels baby who is still warm and gives another dose of acetaminophen from the downstairs bathroom. This mistake can be DEADLY. Double dosing a child on routine fever reducing medication can be a horrible mistake yet happens more commonly then you can imagine.

1. KEEP an old stick of bright red lipstick in the bathroom right next to the bottle of medication.

2. **Whenever you administer the medication write the information on the mirror using your lipstick. It's bright, hard to miss record keeping that may save your child's life. And it usually comes off with a little window cleaner. You might want to check this theory first before writing huge across an heirloom mirror.**

3. **It is also fun to add a little love note to the next person who will be waking up with your little one…i.e. SO GLAD IT IS YOUR TURN, HONEY!**

Who knew bright red lipstick and childcare could be so intricately connected and lifesaving to boot!

When sharing information with your health care practitioner at clinic visits it is also important to keep your commentary as concise as possible. The current world of medicine has enormous demands on a doctor's time. They are often expected to see patients 32-37 hours of a 40-hour workweek. This doesn't allow reasonable time for them to eat lunch or go to the restroom let alone dictating notes about every patient they see, talk with on the phone, read a note about, see an x-ray etc. They also need to call in prescriptions, look over lab and radiology results, phone patients back and answer questions. Many days doctors also do rounds on in-patients, write in charts, dictate letters, keep up with their own Continuing Education Unit's while keeping current with their knowledge about new practices and treatments for certain conditions, new medications on the market and changes in any existing forms of treatments that are discovered to be unsafe. Depending upon their specialty, large groups of physicians also run research studies, lecture at medical institutions and write journals articles or speak about various forms of treatment options they have been working with. So it becomes easier to see why practitioners move quickly in and out of patient rooms. They appreciate when you have thought over your questions in advance and are concise in your description of symptoms. This doesn't mean that your practitioner isn't interested in your comments or willing to stay longer if you have some additional questions it simply means that if the symptoms are straight forward and point directly to a problem it is thoughtful if you are the same. Mutual respect of time and responsibilities is a wonderful way to enhance your relationship with your practitioner and keep in mind how much we appreciate when they respect our time and try not to keep us waiting as well.

Accuracy in health care interactions is one of the most intrical steps to safe and efficient health care delivery. It is vital that everyone involved with your child's welfare has received a concise, precise and global understanding of your child's current issue coupled with their basic medical history. This is the first step towards safe and effect treatment for all of your child's health care needs.

Concept #2
Be Honest

"...a physician can only make a good medical decision based upon the adequate knowledge of what happened."

This seems like an obvious concept when dealing with your doctor. Although when you are in a high stress situation it is so easy to forget details. This concept helps outline how to begin. Then practice this often and it will become a habit that will hopefully see you through the accidents and injuries that are par for the course in parenting. There are 3 specific aspects to this concept:

1. Tell all of your child's symptoms and current medications. Make sure to include all things that are concerning even if you don't know if they are relevant to this specific episode. These things may include: if your child is sleeping

much more recently, or if they are groggy, difficult to wake up, irritable or half awake. Mention if there were accidents or strange occurrences in the child's immediate past. Include past medical problems or illnesses that they have suffered from recently. Also note all medications that they take including multi-vitamin supplements, herbal supplements, or medication that you administered for the current symptoms. Note any current high stress situations that your family may be dealing with as well. Many medical ailments have an emotional component to them, which exacerbates the physical side of the problem.

2. Explain precisely what happened. Note all relevant details including if there was a time

delay before you came to seek medical attention and why. Many parents see their child get a cut or fall and are not sure whether the wound needs to be stitched or not. When they see the laceration again the next day they decide to take the child in but don't mention the time delay. This can lead to serious problems, so don't worry about embarrassment, be honest. This is a firm example of when a physician can only make a good medical decision based upon the adequate knowledge of what happened. If you opt not to provide that information accurately you are not upholding your end of the parent-physician partnership and your child's health will suffer the consequences.

3. Do NOT leave out important details. Having said this, how do you know which are important details and what are things that you could overlook?

Many parents find it difficult to understand how things that seem to be an insignificant detail can turn out to be vital within the medical diagnosis framework. For example, when you go to the doctors for your child's headache, the number of times they need to go to the bathroom or their eating habits may be important. Another child who seems to just stop everything and stare from time to time might seem to be a 'normal' occurrence at your house, but a physician may find that 'habit' to be something worth looking into. There are so many trademark behaviors that you may be used to watching your child do that you simply do not even think about it anymore. But these signs may turn out to be a key symptom that helps assemble all of the pieces of the medical puzzle together for your health care provider.

One way parents (especially first time parents) can begin to pin point these hallmark traits in their own children is to take the time to watch other children your child's age. DO NOT obsess over comparing your child to one particular child. Which is often difficult if you have a niece, nephew or friend with a child similar in age to your own child. So always keep in mind that all children develop at very different rates and it is very normal for your child to vary even a great deal from another child who shares the same age and even a similar genetic make-up. It is often easier to 'watch' children of similar ages in a public area where the children are free to act and respond in ways that they find comfortable. This arena allows you to see their traits while watching your own child's actions and responses in a similar setting. You can see how a variety of children propel themselves around a play structure or what language skills they possess for interaction. How does your child prefer to play; solitary play, close to another child but not really 'with' the other child? By directing other children in their play or interacting back and forth with one or more children? All of these observations helps a parent watch their own child evolve and will offer moments of pride in your child's abilities and also affords the parents a 'birds-eye' view of behaviors you may wish to guide your child through.

One challenge for parents is to stop focusing on what is 'normal' or what other children can or cannot do and start tuning in to your own child. This can only be accomplished by spending large amounts of time with your child, particularly one-on-one time where you are allowing your child to function at their preferred level while showing you things that they enjoy. It is near impossible for a parent to just sit back and observe without intervening and/or correcting. But when you begin to take the control of the situation away from your child you will cease to see your child's preferences and will instead simply substitute in your own wishes and abilities. The gifts of patience and quiet observation are often very difficult to acquire, yet can often be the most vital as a parent. We want to mould and shape our children but find that they wish to be their own sculptors.

As you begin to watch and learn from your child while seeing their behaviors within the framework of age-related milestones that you have learned from observing other children and possibly through research you will develop a sixth sense of what are 'normal developmental tasks and what are variants specific to your child. These unique traits are the things that you may wish to share with your practitioner to gather feedback on or guidance for.

Here is a simple example that may help to make this role of observation and discovery clearer. When our second child was born we were, of course, ecstatic. We held her, loved her and watched her grow in her first couple week's home. At a certain point we began to realize that although she turned her head from side to side and 'watched' us as we entered a room but she seemed to turn more towards the general direction of where we were coming but soon we sensed that she wasn't ever looking directly at us. As the weeks wove into a month we really began to see that she was never actually looking at the toys we would hold over her head. She was very interested in them, but it appeared to be more watching the general direction of the noise but not actually zeroing in on the item. I tried a few things like creeping very quietly into her nursery and seeing if she would respond to me. Or hold a toy over her that didn't make any noise. Did she reach for it, focus on it? Then when she was a couple months old she began to smile towards my face when I spoke, so I thought my suspicions were unfounded and decided not to mention them to my physician. Then we began to notice more marked responses like a strong startle when things would brush the side of her face, it appeared like she didn't see them coming. We quickly discerned that if the toy didn't make noise she was truly not seeing them until they scared her by touching her face.

We finally asked her doctor and pointed out some of our concerns. Our practitioner actually looked relieved that we were noticing something as well. She stated that her first visit when our daughter was fast asleep and she woke her up to do her brief eye exam she was concerned that she wasn't focusing on light or moving objects, but she thought it might have been that our daughter was just disturbed from a sound sleep. But some of the things we were noticing at home were consistent with what she was seeing in the clinic this visit. Our child was blind. We then asked about her ability to smile at us and our physician explained that smiling is actually a neurological response and not necessarily modelled behaviour. A child can smile at you because of comfort and love without ever having seen a

smile. The clues were very subtle for a small infant,

but daily we started seeing more and more things

that didn't fit with our experiences from our other

children. So we did a few easy 'tests' like trying a toy

that didn't make sounds and seeing what his

response was etc. Then we spoke with our

pediatrician and shared our concerns. It was at this

point that we began the long journey of education

and understanding. We progressed through

questioning to information gathering towards

acceptance. Although we were shocked to learn that

our child suffered from a major medical challenge, we

appreciated our practitioner's candid and honest

responses and this openness forged a strong bond

for us to come to them with more questions and

concerns. We were grateful that our practitioner

didn't jump to conclusions and allowed us to share our own concerns before validating them and then expressing concerns of their own.

Another key aspect of the partnership is to avoid blame. It would have been easy for us to get upset with our physician for not mentioning her concerns at the first visit. But that would have been transferring our fear and blame of the unknown onto our care provider because it was convenient and allowed us to openly express some of our anger at the unfairness of our daughter's situation. This would have been very counterproductive, as we need our provider's knowledge and support to learn and understand our changing role and the challenges that would be foreign to us. We understood that although our doctor did have concerns at our last visit she is a person too, and she tried to find other reasons for our daughter's lack of response, knowing that we would return in a couple weeks for another visit, which allowed our daughter another opportunity to show her abilities.

Healthcare providers are people as well as trained practitioners and they also get butterflies, fear and worry when they sense something troubling in their patients. It is oftentimes difficult to overrule that innate yearning to overlook the bad and hope it can be explained away. So they check and double check to make sure that their doubts and fears are founded before passing on the earth shaking news to you as parents. We have learned to truly appreciate the very humanness in our providers and love them all the more for the care, devotion and respect they show their patients.

The honesty in care delivery does not flow in a single direction. It is important that you as parents feel that you have the same respect shown to you by your healthcare team. Parents should feel empowered to challenge a practitioner who does not exemplify this framework. It is also important for parents to accept their role of identification and problem solving when they come upon a medical facility or a practitioner that inhibits a healthy partnership. An example is whenever healthcare providers insist that a parent would leave the room during 'rounds', discussions or care conferences. These are instances where parents not only need to be physically present but should also be a fundamental member of the medical team. It is in these challenging settings when the parent needs to take over the role of educator and let the assembled staff know that they intend to be an essential portion of their child's health care team and are not comfortable with nor will they accept less than a clear partnership within this realm.

One of the best examples I can remember from our own experiences was when our child needed to be placed in a Neonatal Intensive Care facility in a separate hospital and we were told that I could not be transferred over to this facility because of 'political reasons'. We remained adamant that if the health care team was not willing to transfer me I would simply leave AMA(Against Medical Advice). The facility was shocked that I would feel so strongly about wanting to be with my critically ill child. They believed that I should feel comforted to know that he was in a location that could 'adequately' care for him. I was appalled by the fact that any health care facility would believe that a young infant could actually be sufficiently cared for when a parent wasn't present. How could I be part of the health care team when I was not even in attendance when doctor's rounded on him or if critical events happened and I was miles away and without adequate communication. Our baby needed his emotional and psychological needs met as well as his physical ones and in the absence of his only permanent sense of security (i.e. his parent) how could that even be possible.

The other grave loss in a situation similar to this is the idea that upon discharge of the baby, parents really have no knowledge of what medications, treatments, and physical challenges their own child was exposed to during their stay in the NICU. This can be crippling for the parent's confidence when they bring the infant home as well and make it impossible for them to answer even basic health care questions for the rest of the child's life. Critical things like; Has your child ever had this antibiotic before? Has your child ever seized? Was your child on C-PAP, or intubated, if so for how long? Does your child have any allergies? Has your child ever had C-T scan dye before? Or fundamental things like; what kinds of things sooth your child? How does your child like to be held? How much does your child typically eat? The list goes on and on. How can a parent feel secure in their interactions with the child when they have had their role circumvented for such a critical time in their child's life? They no longer feel as if they are the child's primary care giver.

These types of situations that are harmful in establishing the parent's importance as part of the health care delivery team need to be immediately addressed and rectified before they escalate and intensify the endless complications for the parental control and expected parental involvement. If you find yourself in a similar situation as a parent when your physical presence is prohibited you need to make a careful review of the situation, the reasons and purposes behind the proposed separation and your own comfort level. Then you need to advocate for what you feel is in the best interest of your child's well-being. There are rare instances when it may truly be in the best interest of the child to have their parents leave for a period of time. As your child ages, it may become important for your child to possess a degree of privacy in their healthcare team and then the parents need to be ready and willing to transfer some of the responsibility of healthcare partnership off to the child themselves. Though parents will want to make sure that this is done slowly and in stages so that the child can feel confident in their role and responsibilities in this ever-evolving partnership. Even as young as 5 or 6 years old it is helpful to have the child describe their symptoms and feelings to the health care provider. This is the slow process of teaching your child, in your guiding presence, the concepts of this book so that they can slowly assume this role.

Another form of honesty that becomes your responsibility is to share feedback about your personal experiences within the healthcare facility. Lend your time and your knowledge so that the facility can continue to grow and evolve. Each hospital has its own strengths and weakness. No one facility is entirely negative in all of their practices nor is there one exempt from all errors. So share your own insights whether they are individuals whose comfort and guidance was invaluable or a situation that made a difficult time even more stressful. This feedback is instrumental for the facility to know and utilize in the process of eliminating the poor practices and capitalizing on the positive ones. Provide feedback, fill out survey forms, ask for documentation of mistakes, provide praise to individuals and/or departments and write up specific instances of both markedly good and poor care delivery practices. Many facilities have standards that must be followed in the documentation of specific errors, instances or accidents. Recognize that this documentation is vital in the process of continuous improvement that the facility employs to ensure that errors are recorded and learned from. Don't hesitate to offer your candid and honest feedback for providers. Survey forms can be slow to fill out and return, but this information is also vital for facilities that your time and honesty is invaluable for them. Take the time, think about your responses, and be honest and informative. Try to be specific as possible so that problems can be worked out and specific praise can reach its rightful destination.

The creation of your working partnership is a slow and important process, built upon mutual respect, trust, cooperation and shared goals. Parents create the framework of this relationship with their ability to model a strong intention to work conjunctively on building a foundation for this partnership to continue to grow and flourish while practitioners show a wiliness to educate, support and empower the parents in their medical decisions. The parent is primarily responsible for the function of disseminating information to the correct people at the correct time. So they become the first and the most fundamental person in the team of people who will work together to assess, diagnosis and hopefully cure your child. Since most diagnoses are based upon the process of gathering data it is easy to see how imperative honest, concise and timely information is to your child's healthcare delivery.

Concept #3

Ask Questions

"In the 21st century it is vital that you reclaim the knowledge of your medical information."

All of the concepts listed in this book are vital to establishing and maintaining a strong working relationship with your healthcare practitioner, and this one is no different. Yet this concept has a second, equally important reason for being: maintaining your child's good health in conjunction with developing and maintaining a fluency within your own knowledge base. Why is it so important for you to have a strong understanding of the tests, illnesses and medications that your child encounters? Many people have grown up believing that it is their physician's responsibility to keep this information. They leave it to their doctor to remember what medication made them sick or when they had a test or what is the Latin term for whatever is wrong with them. Patient's call to mind old phrases like "What am I paying them for?" "They are the keepers of that information..." "That is why they get the big bucks" Yet in many ways this type of thinking went out with mass transportation and the evolving changes in our health care system. People no longer see a local doctor who birthed them, raised generations of their family members and know their voice when they call. In the 21st century it is vital that you reclaim the knowledge of your own medical information.

In this day and age you and your child will see multiple doctors, move several times in your life span, and travel throughout the country and the world. How do all of these changes affect your child's health coverage? Well, most importantly, you can no longer depend upon someone else to be the gatekeeper to this vital information. You need to have access to all of the past and present medical issues facing your child. The only way to accomplish this is by gleaning this information from your health practitioners. I say this not to imply that your doctor doesn't wish to give you this information but to state that it is your job to inquire about it. You must ask questions, get clarification and learn more about the treatments, procedures, medications and diagnoses facing your child. I know this seems challenging and for many people intimidating, yet many of the strategies are quite simple.

First: Never, Never, Never be afraid to ask questions. Ask for clarification, this may be as simple as stating: "I don't understand, what are you saying?"; This doesn't make you look stupid. Remember from back in the introduction; it is your doctor's job to educate you. So when they tell you your child needs a test, ask the doctor or support staff:

- What is involved in this procedure,

- How can I best prepare my child for it;

  o emotionally

  o physically

- What are all of the steps surrounding the test, before during and after?

It often helps prepare children, if you take the time to talk through a procedure step-by-step with them several times before you reach the facility. Use the same technique as you would for getting them ready for the first day of kindergarten. Tell them all of the information and be honest in your approach. Tell them which parts are going to be painful and tell them that you or the technician will be sure to let them know when the painful parts are coming and when they are over. This relives so much of the child's anxiety by taking away the surprise and fear. You respect your child's feelings by allowing them to process the information in privacy and with ample time to ask questions. What happens if they ask you a question you don't know the answer to? Don't hesitate to call their health care provider to get the answer. By honouring your child's feelings, it helps to assure that they will be informed before the bad part will happen. It also helps to establish a vital sense of trust between you and your child.

We began this process when our children were very young babies. At that point they would be crying and tense through the entire doctor's appointment, always fearful of what would happen to them next. But we insisted upon always being with them and we would always firmly and loudly state (So we could be heard over their screaming) "It is going to hurt, Right Now! Mommy is here with you. I won't leave. You are strong. This will help to make you feel better"; lots of phrases of comfort, love and reassurance. Then we would tell them when it is over and we would never tell them it was ALL over until we were absolutely certain that all of the procedures were completely finished.

After two years of consistently practicing these steps through many horrible procedures, our youngest son was then able to enter clinics without screaming, sits through visits where we are able to hold normal conversations and trusts us to be honest with him about what will happen at medical appointments. He is no longer worried when the doctors do benign things like looking in his ears and listening to his heart. He knows that he can trust the situation and that he will be given fair warning before any 'bad' procedures need to be done. It is also very reasonable for the parent to determine when 'enough is enough' for the day. Young children can only go through so much before they are over stimulated and over whelmed. They need to feel that they have some bit of control over the situation. An easy way to help with this is to offer your child a choice whenever possible. They can choose to have the shot in the right or left arm. They can choose to have the procedure sitting on the chair or in your lap. Simple things like these can give back some of the power in an otherwise powerless situation.

Before each test or procedure make sure to ask your doctor:

1. What is the actual name of the test being performed? (This is good to know in case you need to reference it later to another doctor. It also helps to jar your memory in case your child has recently had the same procedure somewhere else. If this is the case never hesitate to ask if you can just send for the results of the previous test and thus for-go retesting. Most pediatric physicians are happy

to use tests from other facilities to avoid
exposing your child to more discomfort.)

2. Why are we doing this test?

3. What are we looking for with this procedure?

4. How will this change our plan of care? (This
   simply means; what are the doctors planning to
   do differently because of information gathered
   from this test or procedure.) If this will not
   change the plan of care, ask if it is truly
   necessary to even do the test.

5. What are the possible side effects from this
   treatment, procedure, or drug? (Do not be
   offended if your practitioner doesn't know. They
   may need to refer you to a pamphlet,
   pharmacist, or other technologist.)

6. You DO NOT need to know the 'right' question. Just keep asking until you feel confident that you understand. Or simply say that you are uncomfortable making the decision right now and you need some time to process the information before giving an answer.

7. Never hesitate to ask the practitioner to step out of the room and give you and your spouse some time to talk privately before giving your answer. It is near impossible to have an intense discussion about an important decision with an audience. This can also allow you to include your child in the decision making process. Give him/her the opportunity to ask questions and gather information that they may have missed when the grown-ups were talking.

8. Questions for your provider can be as simple as:

     i. Why are we doing this?

     ii. Will it hurt?

     iii. What if we don't feel comfortable doing this now?

     iv. Where can I go to learn more about this?

     v. How long will it take?

     vi. Will my child feel bad after wards? For how long? Is there something I can do to relieve the discomfort?

     vii. Is there someone I can talk to for more information and a better understanding of what will happen?

A little aside about when and/if your practitioner ever states that they don't know or are unsure about an answer to any question you may have.....DO NOT PANIC...this is not the time to run out and find a new doctor because yours just admitted that they don't have all the answers...The most important thing to remember is your practitioner is part of a huge team of healthcare providers each specializing in different aspects of the medical process. It is wonderful when a practitioner can utilize all the members of the healthcare delivery team. In this modern world of medicine it is truly impossible for any one person to understand every aspect of medicine and anyone who attempts to make you believe that they know it all is far more scary then the physician who offers you people to reference for information like side effects of drugs or specifics about how certain procedures will play out.

A large portion of a doctor's training is various ways to reference information. Just like how we learn to use a library, they learn to use the other experts throughout the medical arena in order to better serve their patients. Keep this in mind when you are seeing a general practitioner, family practice physician, nurse practitioner, physician's assistant or internist. These practitioners are all trained specifically to care for the routine ailments and issues of human life and are wonderful practitioners to work with if you enjoy the idea of one doctor seeing all of your family members. But also keep in mind that when you are experiencing symptoms outside of the "normal" or issues that are more intense, long-term or acute, it is often a good time for your general practitioner to send you to one of the many specialists who work specifically with that issue or organ system. This is one of the many things you may need to inquire about on your own, if you wish to follow up with a specialist for confirmation or more information. If you feel that you would like the input of a physician specifically trained in the area of medicine that is affected be sure to speak up to your doctor and ask for a referral and/or a recommendation. I have included a very basic overview of medical specialists in the glossary at the back of the book so that you could have a basic understanding of which specialist addresses what problems and concerns.

Understand that not every symptom needs assessment from a specialist. Each time your child suffers from an ear infection they do not normally need to be seen by an Otorhinolaryngologist (Ear, Nose and Throat Doctor). However, if your child has had 7 ear infections in 5 months and their hearing now seems compromised your practitioner may wish for you to see an ENT doctor to give further input about the continued treatment options and to determine if there is a better way to manage the care. If your physician decides to refer your child make sure to inquire about what is the plan after you have the appointment. Are you supposed to return to your primary care physician or will someone call you to go over the various options in your plan of care? This is an important step as many times you go to the specialist and they close the appointment by saying, "I will give your practitioner a call after I get the test results back." This is when you need to assert yourself and let them know that you wish to play a role in the decision making, so who would be the person for you to contact in order to relay the results and help educate you about your treatment choices.

Occasionally referrals end up in a mutual decision to pursue surgical intervention. For a variety of different reasons, a surgical procedure becomes the best option for the health and well-being of your child. Now the questions for you as parents become that much more important.

SURGICAL PROCEDURES

If you and your practitioner decide that your child needs a surgical procedure performed here are some questions that may help you to better understand the next steps

1. Ask if there is a hospital tour for children and their siblings to take at the facility,

2. Ask if your child can bring along a lovey, stuffed animal or toy.

3. Call the hospital ahead of time and ask if they have any special programs to prepare young children for surgeries.

4. Ask if a parent can come back to the operating room with your child to comfort them as they go off to sleep. If this is not possible, make sure that you take the time to prepare your child well in advance so they understand that they will need to go alone.

5. Ask if the child will be awake when they start the IV or if they can have some relaxing gas beforehand so they don't feel the poke.

6. Ask if you will be with your child as they wake up.

7. Ask if the hospital has a Child Life Department, these are people specifically trained to explain medical procedures, help with comfort measures and provide advocacy services for young children.

8. Many hospitals have set educational programs for children who are undergoing surgical interventions. These are wonderful classes to attend with your child to help them learn about what it is like to have a surgery.

9. Most children need to be NPO(have nothing by mouth) for an extended period of time before a surgical procedure. Make sure to ask when your child needs to begin being NPO. Then

make sure to follow the instructions closely. It is an important safety issue to make sure children really have not ingested anything, including the water to take a med or brush your teeth before a surgery.

10.   If your child has unique dietary needs, make sure to let your practitioner know. If your child is still on formula or breast feeding let the staff know when you are discussing NPO status. Also if your child is diabetic make sure to discuss dietary and insulin needs long before the day of the surgery.

Chronic or Complicated Diagnosis:

If your child is diagnosed with a chronic condition or disorder, besides gathering medical information you may also wish to learn more about what supportive services are out there to aid your child and help your entire family better cope with the challenges that lay ahead. The process of diagnosis is often best understood and accepted when it is eased into like walking slowly into the ocean on a very gradual beach. You get a chance to grow accustom to the changing temperature of the water and feel your way over the sandy beach to let your body and mind adjust to the changes. The discouraging reality is that diagnoses seldom happen in this way. Most diagnoses have to be quick and direct. In these instances make sure to allow yourself and your child more time to process the information during and after the event.

When someone tells you that your child is deaf, blind, profoundly disabled, gravely or chronically ill; it is life changing, mind-boggling and simply an overwhelming experience. Expect that you and your family will go through a full grieving process. Time, compassion, control and a supportive environment are all hallmarks to surviving and thriving through a grief cycle. Children experience grief as well. Be prepared to offer your child an environment rich in compassion, acceptance and understanding. Watch for signs of interruptions in the normal grief cycle. Any marked changes in your child's normal behaviors that do not resolve within a short period of time need to be shared with your practitioner and addressed immediately. Never underestimate the impact of emotional health upon the healing of your child's physical disorders.

If you find that your family is facing multiple stressors that are complicating your medical care, family structure or global healthcare delivery ask for a referral to Social Services. This is a group of wonderful practitioners who specialize in understanding the family support network and what are things that can be done to help strengthen your family's structure. They also can find resources for some of the more basic yet fundamental needs like where to stay if you are traveling from afar, or how to deal with family and friends etc. Social Services can also help you to interact with your child's school systems, if your child is going to be hospitalized and needs to miss school for any period of time. There are often good resources to keep your child up to date on their schooling and keep their mind active while their body heals

There are also resources to help gather information and further long term support for siblings, extended family and friends if the diagnosis will have long-term or far reaching impacts on your families' daily lives. They have valuable networks of other health professionals they can draw upon to help with directing you and your family towards solutions for a large variety of different challenges.

There are also countless support groups out there of parents facing some of the same things that you will go through. Do not try to travel the road alone, reach out for help and understanding. I believe that no one should ever have to reinvent the wheel. Learn from others, lean on others, share their knowledge and ease your path through their insight.

Concept #4
Leave With a Plan

"Education is the key to understanding, confidence and empowerment."

    As your visit begins to come to a close and you feel confident that you have been heard, feel educated and were empowered to make decisions that sit comfortably within the framework of your family's values and priorities. You now are preparing to leave your appointment. In order to go home and continue in your role as an essential part of your child's health care delivery team you must walk home with both; knowledge and power!

Knowledge:

- You must have a firm understanding about what is wrong with your child.

Power:

- You must also feel confident in the role you are being asked to play in supporting and promoting good health for your child.

- You must feel confident that you can manage the ongoing care and facilitate healing?

- And you must have a firm plan about when or if you should return with your child for a follow-up appointment?

Although you may feel comfortable with this limited information as you leave the appointment you may be doing yourself a great disservice if you walk away from the appointment now. Depending upon your background and your life experiences you may be able to take your child home with this limited information and 9 times out of 10 have no complications and experience no frustration from your incomplete information. You may in-fact be reading this thinking, "What more is there to know?" But problems arise when you go home and some times in the middle of the night (because complications always occur like clockwork, right after the clinic closes and your resources have just gone home to their own families.) So now your plan, which you felt comfortable with, just crumbled like stale bread. Your child broke out in a rash, spiked a fever, started throwing up, didn't get better after many days on the medication, or a whole host of other possibilities that always seem to crop up when you least expect them. Now what are your options? You sit there rocking your precious little one in the middle of the night wondering how all of your well-laid plans of good health and clear sailing just went up in smoke. The real issue in this scenario was simply an incomplete plan, and if you have been lucky enough to never have an issue backfire so far don't bank on your luck forever. Sooner or later you are going to take your little one home from an appointment with a 'well-laid' plan and find out that you didn't even begin to have all of the answers to your questions.

So what are some of the missing questions?

- What is the diagnosis? Have you ever heard your provider tell you it was myelitisiwneoruhafhdfoi...? Shook your head, took your child home, then he or she got worse in the night, you take them back to the ER or Urgent Care the new doctor asks you about your previous visit (because, of course, the notes aren't on your child's chart yet) and you look at them and say "AHHHHH, He has something wrong....Look we have medication." Then you want to kick yourself for not having written down what your original practitioner said?

- What are signs to watch for that may mean the condition is worsening? (You often assume that you will recognize these signs. Like a bright red flag, which will pop up saying.."Things are worse take her/him back in." But this seldom happens. It is usually a combination of several vague signs, which makes the decision murky as to whether this symptom requires another visit or should you just call in. Ask for clarification. A common symptom that can mean the condition is worsening is a sleepy, lethargic child. But many parents think this is a good sign that the child is resting and "getting better." Be careful a very sleepy child, especially one that is very difficult to wake up can be a very alarming sign.

- Is it safe for your child to resume normal activities? Many times it is normal or expected that your child can do whatever they feel comfortable doing. But there are rare instances when your health care provider may feel that rest, quiet play or complete bed rest are the more appropriate way to encourage healing.

- Is it safe for your child to interact with other children? If not; for how long should they be kept separate? This is a vital question. As your child begins to encounter multiple children in their social circle you will immediately see the instance of illness double. This is often because parents do not understand disease processes or in some cases they don't use common sense in deciding when to bring their children to social functions or to daycare settings.

- Who should I call if the medicine makes him sick, gives her a rash or seems to be making the symptoms worse?

- How long until we see some of the symptoms lessening?

- What should we do if this medication doesn't seem to be helping?

- How long should we wait before returning to the clinic if the symptoms don't get better?

This knowledge gives you the power to help make better parenting decisions. It will also help you to assess various situations, both now and in the future as to their emergent nature and in other cases, will help you to judge good follow-up practices. The more information you collect, the more control you have in the typical, uncontrollable life of a parent. View these answers as tools in your parenting handbag. Each of them will help you to review symptoms, assess reactions and obtain important information before you make decisions. A big part of parenting is making split second decisions based on limited information and with high emotional investment. Which is, of course, the essential Catch 22. However, if you use this concept in achieving a formulated plan before leaving the clinic you will help to augment the challenges that are weighing down your decision-making process. You can now be free to make a

confident, informed decision.

For Parents of Children with Special Needs

"A ground swell of support may not take away the pain and fear but it can make sure you never feel alone in your trepidation or isolated in your needs."

Parents with children who have chronic, acute, unique or multi-faceted diagnoses are faced with submersion into the healthcare community. There can be an enormous amount of 'culture-shock'. You realize quickly that they speak a different language, communicate in abbreviations and acronyms, wear different clothes and are always in a rush. Then you have the challenge of decoding what they are telling you. Processing the information in a timely fashion. Advocating for your child in an intimidating atmosphere of medical knowledge and then making what may be a life-changing decision in a very short period of time. Often we wonder if it would be helpful to have had advanced warning that this was happening so we could have planned, learned more, or prepared ourselves. But you quickly comprehend that when a diagnosis is made and the cogs of the medical world begin to churn you are swept into a whirlpool of emotions, decisions and turmoil that nothing could have prepared you for. You realize that you were glad you got to hold onto 'normal' as long as possible and you now wish you would have appreciated that quiet, sedate little life a lot more.

If you have not had the chance to read the section on chronic illnesses in Concept #3, Asking questions section, I encourage you to page back and read those pieces carefully.

PEOPLE TO PEOPLE RESOURCES

This is just a small listing of some 'in-person' items that will hopefully generate ideas, or questions. Often the only reason why you didn't receive the support or information is because you simply didn't know to ask. The other purpose behind generating interest is spreading great ideas across the country and around the world. Never hesitate to take a good idea that you hear happening and inquire about the possibility of developing something similar in your own community or clinic. Many clinics value the input and ideas of parents. They recognize that parents are consumers and are often the best grass roots movements for new areas of growth. It can be life changing to feel support when you desperately need it and parents of disabled children are usually an incredibly compassionate bunch. The big hope is that no one goes through the same struggles and failures that 'we' had to face. But disabled parents are often an exhausted and overwhelmed bunch as well so we need to spread our ideas so that no one has to 'reinvent the wheel'. **A ground swell of support may not take away the pain and fear but it can make sure you never feel alone in your trepidation or isolated in your needs.**

- **Handouts and Flyers at your clinic:** This is often your first line of resources. The doctor comes in, tells you that your child has a specific diagnosis and then refers you to the clinic staff who will hand you a few flyers about the disease. Make sure to look over the flyers and/or pamphlets. Even if it is a simple one-sheet pamphlet often times at the bottom there will be a list of several websites or a phone number to call...'with further questions.' These are great places to begin your investigation.

- **Patient Education Departments:** Many mid to large sized facilities now have specific education departments. If the clinic itself doesn't have one, often the hospital that it is affiliated with will. Sometimes education departments are a small room with a single person. Don't be put off by this. All you need is one knowledgeable person who knows where to go for resources and accurate information. One education department we worked with was in the basement of an inner city hospital with 2 people, several file cabinets, and a few computers. But those two people really knew where to find accurate timely information. One facility had a small lounge called the Parent Resource Room. Besides having comfortable chairs and free coffee (always a treat for parents who are doing the long sleepless haul as inpatients) they offered a wonderful service: parents could come in, give their first name, their room number and the disease, disorder, treatment or surgery they were looking for more information on. Then within a day the education people would do all the research for them and package it in a folder that is then delivered up to their child's room complete with tabs and an index of other resources. What SERVICE! If your facility lacks for educational resources, start asking around, sometimes patient interest can generate positive change.

- **Social Services:** This is the Number One best resource for parents of long term chronic issues because they can help you to look at your entire family structure and assist in greater ways than just a short-term one-time fix. They are great resources for explaining how others have handled the same situation. For instance, many families who have children recently diagnosed with disabilities, face several of the same challenges... Like:

How can I juggle time off work to be available for my child and still be financially responsible? There are often no great answers to this question but many people are creative in their attempt to solve this problem so don't 'start from square one' build on someone else's great idea. Ask for more information about the Family Medical Leave Act. I put a copy of the federal law in the index section of this book just so you wouldn't have to hunt for a general reference. This is the federal law that stipulates a 12 week leave from work without any worry about loss of job. Make sure to review the information provided or visit the website to note the stipulations surrounding this mandate. Also note that this is unpaid leave.

Are there local hotels that offer hospital rates or weekly rates? Sometimes the hospital keeps a list of different lodgings who have discounted rates or offer special bonuses for families with children who are inpatient for long periods of time. One of the best benefits that hotels can offer to families is free laundry facilities. We have a hotel we routinely use that are wonderful and they even offer a free hotel shuttle to and from the hospital at any hour of the day or night so you don't need to hunt and pay for parking.

There is also a hospital in St. Paul MN: Gillette Children's Hospital, who has a Ronald McDonald House located within the hospital itself. They serve free meals for families each night. They also have several beautiful hotel-like rooms right there on-site where you can stay for free. It is truly amazing.

Make sure to ask the social worker about rooming in as well. One of us always slept right in the room with our child whenever they were an inpatient and many facilities will find a place for the other parent to sleep in-house as well. But if you have other children or are staying for an extended period it is nice to have a place to go to switch off getting a real night's sleep.

What happens should you do if your child needs to miss a great deal of school for a lengthy hospital stay? Your social worker usually has a routine that they follow with this one. They will often work closely with your home district or the hospital will offer some type of tutoring services that will then be sent back to your home district upon completion of your stay. They will usually work closely with you and your child to make sure that the work is not too taxing or overwhelming for your child depending upon their physical state. But if you are not approached and you feel concerned about how much school your child is missing or you think that the intellectual stimulation would be a good distraction from the monotony of the hospital stay, never hesitate to ask your Social Worker about what the options are.

Are there other families out there that we can connect with to learn from and be mentored by? Sometimes health facilities have a commons areas or parent lounges that are somewhat designed for facilitating interaction between parents that will hopefully lead to mutual support and information exchange. But if you don't find a structured area, the play areas will often serve the same purpose. It can be a good relief to talk, vent and share with someone who is experiencing many of the same struggles and emotions. If you don't find a resource within the hospital setting, or for when you return home, don't hesitate to ask about outside parent support groups, educational groups or parent-to-parent organizations. There are many parent advocacy groups that have trained families who are matched with newly diagnosed families. They offer practical advice, support and caring interaction. Some churches have resources for parent support groups as well. Don't hesitate to ask around and make sure to find a family that is a good match for your needs and values.

Although you will have endless questions and your Social Worker will desperately try to help you find resources, keep in mind that in many instances their hands are politically or financially tied. But always ask; there are many programs out there for families who need a few meals while they stay in the hospital or to help alleviate some small financial stress a family may be experiencing. There will be no amount of help that can take away from having a very sick child, but if some of your other stresses are minimized this support may offer you the simple luxury of focusing on your child's health.

- **Pediatric Specific Facilities:** If your child is looking at a long hospital stay or multiple admissions over a period of time, there is no substitute for a facility that specializes in pediatrics. It is wonderful to find a site that has a total focus on children and their special needs. It is an amazing feeling for parents when each department has your child as their number one focus. Pediatric facilities have the luxury to offer lab, radiology, surgery and dietary departments that specialize in family friendly focused services. The facilities often have multiple playrooms that are staffed by Child Family Life staff who can customized play to suit your child's needs and abilities. They may be able to help your child to better understand the procedures and treatments they are going through. The best part about child-specific facilities is the knowledge that everyone there loves kids and wants to make your child's experience a positive one.

- **Local School System:** Your local school system can be another great resource of possibilities. Depending upon your child's long-term prognosis the district may work with you to develop a specific educational plan that focuses on your child's needs, abilities, and healthcare schedule. Even if your child does not need an Individualized Educational Plan(IEP) or Family Educational Plan(FEP) the district may be able to work to help you find resources or give your ideas for shorter-term solutions. Usually the key contact people are located within the Special Education Department. Each district usually has a physical therapist, occupational therapist, speech pathologist, special education instructor and/or adaptive professionals on staff. So if your child is going to have compromised abilities for a short period of time or an extended one these professionals are willing to work with you and help you find the easiest way to transition your child back into the school setting. They may also be consulted to help the other children to understand and communicate with your child. One example of simple yet very helpful information we received: one time we mentioned, by chance, to our physical therapist that our son has trouble doing stretches because of the pulling and strain, but he loves to swim. So she did some searching and found a local hotel who was willing to let her do PT during the days with our son in their pool for a nominal amount each visit. We now just turned a usually stressful time and transformed into a time of beneficial fun. We then realized that because of our son's stiff muscles he didn't move around enough to keep his body temperature up for any period of time in the pool so he would end up shivering and blue lipped after an hour physical therapy session. So with some investigation through the catalogues that she receives, our physical therapist was able to find a very reasonably priced 'wet suit' that helped him to maintain his body temp so he could better tolerate the temperatures. Now he enjoys his stretching and they get a lot more work done with each visit.

- **Parent Support Groups:** These can be listed in the yellow pages, on line, in your newspaper community calendar sections and through churches. They are wonderful places to talk, gain support, understanding and connect with other families who are experiencing grief, emotional struggles and times of crisis. These families hold a wealth of knowledge about the ins and outs of caring for a child with special needs. They also work as great resources to learn about future problems you may be able to proactively address. It is always so much more effective to plan for issues rather than simply reacting to them. It is also a fun place to share your everyday joys, gain support and hear insights with others who share the same hills and valleys that you do.

Support groups are also great resources for other fun programs or activities designed for families facing medical challenges. They can be a font of new avenues to try, new adventure to explore and new people to meet and enjoy.

Nurse line/Case Management worker for your Health Insurance Company: More and more insurance companies are sponsoring their own nurse help lines. You may find these resources to be helpful or you may find that your questions are too specific or in depth. We found that our specialty doctor's offices were often the easier route for answers. They usually have a nurse you can talk to and they can answer the more specific questions about your child's particular ailment and how your doctor would like you to address it. Case Management Nurses through your health Insurance

Company are also becoming more popular. These individuals are assigned to follow complicated patients through their health care journey. They will usually call you to initiate contact and then will continue to phone you on a regular basis to see how your child is doing and to help coordinate the care for your child.

Parent Advocacy Services: I mentioned these earlier, but will elaborate a bit more. Spend some time to look for these groups or organizations. You may find some at your local level or look to nationally sponsored agencies. These can be wonderful resources that guide you through the process of advocating for your child. They are usually made up of trained Parent Professionals who have been in shoes similar to yours. They are there to simply help you navigate the very confusing world of disabilities.

They can educate you, offer resources, empower you and advocate for you and your child. They usually are free or carry a very nominal charge. Yet always remember that when your life finally finds a balance the best service you can offer them is your willingness to mentor another family through the process. Our communities are always looking for volunteers to help fellow families navigate the turbulent waters of chronic illness and disability.

- **Camps and Conferences:** Many common chronic conditions have camps specifically designed for children who suffer from this particular disorder. There are also general camps for children with disabilities or medical challenges. As your child become more accepting of their disorder they will often find comfort in learning that others have walked this road. They can gain a great deal of perspective meeting other children who face the same daily struggles that they do. It is a wonderful environment for children to learn how to answer questions about their disease, or interact with children who are blunt or rude.

Adult educational conferences serve this same purpose for parents. We found a wealth of conferences through our state public school system website they are often meant for educators of special needs children but much of the information can be valuable for parents as well. Parent Advocacy Programs are often strong resources for keeping parents up-to-date about when and where these conferences are. Always look for information about scholarships or grants that may help you afford these sometimes-pricey conferences.

- **Parent Advisory Groups:** Many healthcare facilities have advisory boards made up of parents who utilize their facility and can now guide them in the process of continuous improvement. These groups provide valuable insight for facilities to look at improvement and change. This is a great place for parents to join in the forum to work towards improvement for families who will be facing similar struggles in the future.

Computer Resources

- **General Websites:** It helps to start your search with a larger site, like a specific hospital, disease specific website etc. and then click upon links available to learn more and more. There is so much information out there, that it can be a bit overwhelming. I found it helpful to use the library or educational department to aid in directing this so you can help find accurate information. If you don't have help available always start with websites that you know to be very reputable. Like: The American Academy of Pediatrics, a children's hospital from a large metropolitan area, a parenting website etc. These are great places to begin your search.

- **Websites for Disease Specific Information:** One of the easiest ways to begin your investigation is to do a search for your specific disease name. Many of the common childhood diseases host their own websites and have great informational and educational aspects to their site.

They may also list local support groups, area

events, chat areas or places for further resources.

Never hesitate to click on links. I could spend

hours going through informational websites. They

have a wealth of information and insight that can

be very useful for parents as their child accepts

and assimilates to their new diagnosis.

- **Website Generating Medical Information:**

There are many websites out there that offer

'laymen's' explanations for medical diagnoses. They

often try to take the place of a health care

professional in diagnosing and offering treatment

options. This can be very tempting for parents to use

because they are nervous about symptoms their child

may be experiencing and it may be after hours, hard

to get an appointment or more nerve wrecking to go to a clinic setting. Be very careful in your use of these sites. Remember that a healthcare professional uses an intricate set of assessment tools coupled with a vast background of knowledge and experience when diagnosing and treating a patient. They never look at one isolated symptom, or zero in a single possibility. They assess, explore, ask questions, gather data and then use all of this information to help them make a decision based upon multiple criteria. These websites are not meant to be used in place of a visit with a health practitioner. Yet more and more often patients are doing too many self-assessments based upon a single session with an internet site. Without the ability to look deeper, view all of the options and pursue testing to back up a diagnosis, there is no way that anyone should come to a conclusion based upon such limited information. It becomes easy to understand how misleading this information can be when you realize that there are hundreds of diagnoses whose main symptoms are; stomach upset, tiredness, and feeling of general unease. So be careful when choosing to utilize a website to assess anyone's medical symptoms.

A good use of these websites is to gather a working definition for current diagnosis, or read through the layman's explanation. It can also help parent's process the information that has already been told to them by their healthcare staff. It can be very beneficial to hear and see the information so that you feel that you have a firm understanding of the disease your child is being diagnosed with. The information you read through may help you to formulate questions that serve to heighten your understanding and clarify your child's future experiences with this disorder. Be careful of any predictions that may appear on a website. Make sure that you clarify these with your practitioner before assuming that they apply to your child's specific case.

Another way to utilize the information provided on a medical website is to learn more about tests and procedures that are used to diagnosis or treat the specific disorder that your child has. Make sure to always inquire with your practitioner about whether this test or treatment will be used for your child and what the risks/benefits to each option are. Then you can achieve a deeper understanding of the days and months ahead. You may then use this information to help prepare your child and your extended family.

- **Websites of Periodicals for Disabled Families:** There are many magazines, and newsletters out there directed specifically for families with disabled children. The first place to begin looking is in the racks at your doctor's offices, pediatric hospitals and parent resource rooms. These range from disease specific periodicals all the way through parenting magazines designed for parents of special needs children or exceptional parents. These magazines provide a myriad of practical information, nation-wide resources and valuable candid accounts from families themselves. It can be a regular shot of hope and inspiration for families who are greatly in need.

All of these resources are meant to augment the information you are gathering from your own healthcare staff. Since all families are different, you may find that it is more helpful for you to hear a first-hand account from another family or you may prefer to read articles in the privacy of your own home. You will also find that at different times during the entire process of hearing, thinking, feeling and acceptance of a medical diagnosis you may need to acquire your information in different ways so that you are better able to understand and manage it. Be kind to yourself and explore all of the possibilities so that you can find accurate information and the optimal way to acquire it. Information for a family with a disabled child is a veritable lifeline that guides you through a confusing and often dark world. Remember that the more you know the better you are equipped to care for yourself and your child.

Conclusion

"A practitioner who you trust, respect and have a strong working partnership is one of the most important relationships that any parent can have."

Parenting is the pinnacle of personal accomplishment wrapped in the most distressing of self-examination and recriminations. All parents struggle with the pendulum swing from extreme joy and fulfilment; back towards guilt and self-doubt. Health care issues intensify these feelings for parents because it is one of the rare times when you cannot come up with the answer through your own thoughts, values and feelings. Most parents face times each day where they think; "I wish someone would just tell me the right answer to this parenting dilemma and I would be happy to just follow that path instead of having to always weigh the risks, benefits, and experience all of the guilt." Although parents may feel this on occasion, most would not actually be comfortable with this situation because in reality they do want to be the primary participant in raising their child. So when a parent must seek outside information and expertise in a medical decision, it is a personal struggle for them to accept this information into their own vernacular and evaluate it, without challenging the notion of being forced to have a stranger take such an active role in helping to 'parent' their child. There are many healthcare concepts specifically addressed to help train medical students in this 'Family-Centered' form of patient care delivery. It is a privilege to be asked by a parent to accept the responsibility of joining the family system in such an intimate and important way. Health care providers need to learn appropriate techniques in fostering this partnership so that they are able to provide parents with this vital education while empowering them to accept the role of primary decision maker in a medically guided way. This helps to continue to facilitate the parental role that will be vital to the child's well-being long after the physician is not even a memory for the child. The concepts in this book were designed to help guide parents through their roles within this partnership while also educating them about their personal responsibilities. As in all areas of medicine parents need to be the primary advocate for their child's needs and welfare. It can be intimidating to address these concerns with people who are academically superior in this one realm, but parents simply need to remember their role and its continuing importance to the life- long health of their child.

These four concepts are also meant to open doors of thought for families and empower them while acknowledging the incredible importance of the parent's role in their child's medical team. They do not, however, address specific instances or concerns that individual parents may face nor do they mean to provide medical answers for parents facing dilemmas in their child's physical health. These concepts can never take the place of a physician, they are in fact here to recognize the significance of having a strong practitioner on your side, as a parent. A practitioner who you trust, respect and have a strong working partnership is one of the most important relationships that any parents can have. Cultivate the relationship. Respect it. Celebrate it! Practitioners can be a link for parents to their own sense of reassurance and peace of mind.

My family embraced this belief after a great deal of searching and many hours of communication over years of time. We now have a team of health care providers who are vital parts of our extended family. We care about them, respect them and value their important role in our children's health and in the emotional and physical well-being of our entire family structure. We cannot stress enough the value that we set in our relationships with our providers but we also recognize that this responsibility is a decidedly two-way street. We have encouraged and cultivated these relationships in countless ways throughout the years. We were greatly encouraged by the response of our daughter when she was about 5 years old; after years of spending 20+ hours a week in the company of our providers to care for her disabled sibling, we asked her why she thought we spent so much time with doctors….her response was simply, "Because they are our friends and we love them" I guess for us that really says it all.

This healthy, vital, working partnership is the key to your child's good health! Look to them for information, support, encouragement and collaboration.

Good Luck and Good Health to you and your family….

Glossary

This is a brief listing, in 'layman's term' of each medical specialty and basic areas in which they specialize. For a more complete listing look on medical websites or in a medical dictionary/encyclopaedia.

Anesthesiology: *Administers medications to control the loss of sensation during surgery or traumatic procedures, Works with pain management*

Cardiology: *Works with conditions or diseases of the heart and blood vessels*

Child Life Specialist: *champions your child's need to interact, learn and cope at their developmental level. They work with your child through play, reading, talking, imagining and art to help them to understand and assimilate what is happening in their world.*

Dermatology: *deals with diseases and disorders of the skin*

Emergency Medicine: *Stablizes patients in critical conditions*

Endocrinology: *Works with diseases of the endocrine glands examples: thyroid, pituitary gland etc.*

ENT: *see Otorhinolaryngology*

Genetics: diagnoses and manages the care of people experiencing disorders that are of a genetic nature.

Family Practice: general practitioner who can care for patients of all ages. Helps to promote wellness and does well baby and child checks.

Gastroenterology: handles disease of the stomach, small intestine, large intestine and all the organs that contribute to this system; liver, pancreas, and gall bladder.

Gerontology: deals with diseases and disorders of elderly people

Gynecology: Deals with disease and disorders of the female reproductive tract

Internal Medicine: Handles all diseases and disorders of individuals over the age of 18.

Neonatology: manages the care of babies facing critical conditions in the first few weeks of life.

Neurology: deals with diseases and disorders of the brain, spine, and nervous system. Manages the care of patients with seizures disorders.

Obstetrics: Manages the care of pregnant women through delivery.

Occupational Therapist: this professional works with your child's fine motor movements and helps *your child to develop daily living skills with 'regular' utensils or they may enhance your child's ability to learn by using specialized equipment. Some of the skills they focus on are; daily living skills, writing, drawing, dressing, eating, daily cares, and basic hygiene skills. They may also help to look at various forms of assistive technology to help your child achieve their optimal success.*

Occupational Therapists may come to your home or work with your child in the school system. Health care facilities also employed OT's to work with children while they are in the hospital or as outpatients.

Oncology: *deals with the diagnosis and treatment of all tumors or issues relate to managing the care of patients with cancer.*

Ophthalmology: *handles diseases and disorders of the eye.*

Orthopedics: *deals with disease and disorders with the muscular or skeletal systems.*

Otorhinolaryngology: *deals with diseases or disorders of the ear, nose or throat.*

Pathology: *Studies samples taken from organs, tissues or cells and notes changes or areas of concern.*

Pediatrics: *deals with diseases and disorders specific to children under the age of 18 years old, sometimes they will care for children up to the age of 21.*

Perinatology: *manages the fetal growth and development in high-risk pregnancies or pregnancies of multiple births.*

Pulmonology: *Handles diseases and disorders of the lungs and airway. They are also often involved in managing children in the intensive care unit*

Physiatrist: *works with rehabilitating people, or managing issues of movement and physical medicine.*

Physical Therapist: *Helps the kids with movement, stretching, and gross motor development. They often will come to your home or work with the child in the school system, but health care facilities also employ PT's to work with children while they are in the hospital or as outpatients.*

Plastic Surgery: *deals with corrective surgery designed to repair injured or malformed areas of the body.*

Proctology: *Deals specifically with disease of the lower intestinal tract.*

Psychiatry: *handles diseases or disorders of the mind.*

Radiology: *reads x-rays and other radiographic materials to aid in diagnosis, uses radiation to treat diseases.*

Social Worker: *offers information and support by guiding your family through the challenges of hospitalization, chronic diagnosis or complicated medical outcomes.*

Speech Pathologist: *helps to capitalize on your child's ability to communicate. They may help with sign language, augmentative forms of communication, computer assisted technology or devises that will help your child to interact and communicate with the outside world.*

Sports Medicine: *works with the prevention and treatment of injuries directly related to sports*

Surgery: *performs surgery to treat injuries and disease, or correct specific issues.*

Thoracic Surgery: *Performs surgery for areas related specifically to issues concerning the lungs, heart or chest cavity.*

Urology: deals with diseases and disorders specific to the organs of the urinary tract including; the kidneys, bladder, ureter and urethra.

FAMILY MEDICAL LEAVE ACT: For a more extensive listing
of the entire law see... www.dol.gov/esa/whd/fmla

Definition of the Family Medical Leave Act

  (a) The Family and Medical Leave Act of 1993 (FMLA or
Act) allows
``eligible'' employees of a covered employer to take job-
protected,
unpaid leave, or to substitute appropriate paid leave if
the employee
has earned or accrued it, for up to a total of 12
workweeks in any 12
months because of the birth of a child and to care for the
newborn
child, because of the placement of a child with the
employee for
adoption or foster care, because the employee is needed
to care for a
family member (child, spouse, or parent) with a serious
health
condition, or because the employee's own serious health
condition makes
the employee unable to perform the functions of his or
her job (see
Sec. 825.306(b)(4)). In certain cases, this leave may be
taken on an
intermittent basis rather than all at once, or the employee
may work a
part-time schedule.

  (b) An employee on FMLA leave is also entitled to have
health
benefits maintained while on leave as if the employee had
continued to
work instead of taking the leave. If an employee was
paying all or part
of the premium payments prior to leave, the employee
would continue to

pay his or her share during the leave period. The employer may recover
its share only if the employee does not return to work for a reason
other than the serious health condition of the employee or the
employee's immediate family member, or another reason beyond the
employee's control.

(c) An employee generally has a right to return to the same position
or an equivalent position with equivalent pay, benefits and working
conditions at the conclusion of the leave. The taking of FMLA leave
cannot result in the loss of any benefit that accrued prior to the start
of the leave.

(d) The employer has a right to 30 days advance notice from the
employee where practicable. In addition, the employer may require an
employee to submit certification from a health care provider to
substantiate that the leave is due to the serious health condition of
the employee or the employee's immediate family member. Failure to
comply with these requirements may result in a delay in the start of
FMLA leave. Pursuant to a uniformly applied policy, the employer may
also require that an employee present a certification of fitness to
return to work when the absence was caused by the employee's serious
health condition (see Sec. 825.311(c)). The employer may delay restoring
the employee to employment without such certificate relating to the

health condition which caused the employee's absence.
[60 FR 2237, Jan. 6, 1995; 60 FR 16383, Mar. 30, 1995]

The Purpose of the Family Medical Leave Act:

(a) FMLA is intended to allow employees to balance their work and
family life by taking reasonable unpaid leave for medical reasons, for
the birth or adoption of a child, and for the care of a child, spouse,
or parent who has a serious health condition. The Act is intended to
balance the demands of the workplace with the needs of families, to
promote the stability and economic security of families, and to promote
national interests in preserving family integrity. It was intended that
the Act accomplish these purposes in a manner that accommodates the
legitimate interests of employers, and in a manner consistent with the
Equal Protection Clause of the Fourteenth Amendment in minimizing the
potential for employment discrimination on the basis of sex, while
promoting equal employment opportunity for men and women.

(b) The enactment of FMLA was predicated on two fundamental
concerns--the needs of the American workforce, and the development of
high-performance organizations. Increasingly, America's children and
elderly are dependent upon family members who must spend long hours at
work. When a family emergency arises, requiring workers to attend to

seriously-ill children or parents, or to newly-born or adopted infants,
or even to their own serious illness, workers need reassurance that they
will not be asked to choose between continuing their employment, and
meeting their
personal and family obligations or tending to vital needs at home.

   (c) The FMLA is both intended and expected to benefit employers as
well as their employees. A direct correlation exists between stability
in the family and productivity in the workplace. FMLA will encourage the
development of high-performance organizations. When workers can count on
durable links to their workplace they are able to make their own full
commitments to their jobs. The record of hearings on family and medical
leave indicate the powerful productive advantages of stable workplace
relationships, and the comparatively small costs of guaranteeing that
those relationships will not be dissolved while workers attend to
pressing family health obligations or their own serious illness.

This is the 6 x 9 Basic Template. Paste your manuscript into this template or simply start typing. Delete this text prior to use.